Complications
in Anesthesia

Section Editors

JOHN L. ATLEE, MD
Professor of Anesthesiology
Department of Anesthesiology
Medical College of Wisconsin
Milwaukee, Wisconsin

BRENDA A. BUCKLIN, MD
Associate Professor of Anesthesiology
Department of Anesthesiology
University of Colorado Health Sciences Center
Denver, Colorado

MARK A. CHANEY, MD
Associate Professor of Anesthesiology
Department of Anesthesia and Critical Care
University of Chicago Pritzker School of Medicine
Chicago, Illinois

DONN M. DENNIS, MD, FAHA
Joachim S. Gravenstein, MD, Professor of Anesthesiology
Department of Anesthesiology
University of Florida College of Medicine
Gainesville, Florida
Vice President-Pharmacology, ARYx Therapeutics, Inc.
Santa Clara, California

JOHN ELLIS, MD
Professor of Anesthesiology
Department of Anesthesia and Critical Care
University of Chicago Pritzker School of Medicine
Chicago, Illinois

JOEL M. GUNTER, MD
Professor of Clinical Anesthesia and Pediatrics
Department of Anesthesia
University of Cincinnati School of Medicine
Attending Anesthesiologist
Department of Anesthesia
Children's Hospital Medical Center
Cincinnati, Ohio

ROSEMARY HICKEY, MD
Professor and Program Director
Department of Anesthesiology
University of Texas Health Science Center at San Antonio
San Antonio, Texas

BRIAN M. ILFELD, MD
Associate Professor
Department of Anesthesia
University of California, San Diego
San Diego, California

DONALD A. KROLL, MD, PHD
Staff Anesthesiologist
Department of Surgery
Veterans Affairs Medical Center
Biloxi, Mississippi

TERRI G. MONK, MD
Professor
Department of Anesthesiology
Duke University Medical Center
Durham, North Carolina

TIMOTHY E. MOREY, MD
Associate Professor of Anesthesiology
Department of Anesthesiology
University of Florida College of Medicine
Gainesville, Florida

MICHAEL J. MURRAY, MD, PHD
Professor of Anesthesiology and Chair
Department of Anesthesiology
Mayo Clinic College of Medicine
Jacksonville, Florida

NADER D. NADER, MD
Associate Professor of Anesthesiology, Surgery and
    Pathology
State University of New York at Buffalo School of
    Medicine
Buffalo, New York

MICHAEL F. O'CONNOR, MD
Associate Professor
Department of Anesthesia and Critical Care
University of Chicago Pritzker School of Medicine
Chicago, Illinois

KERRI M. ROBERTSON, MD
Associate Clinical Professor of Anesthesiology
Chief, General, Vascular, High-Risk Transplant and Surgical
    Critical Care Medicine Division
Chief, Transplant Services
Duke University School of Medicine
Department of Anesthesiology
Durham, North Carolina

SCOTT R. SPRINGMAN, MD
Professor
Departments of Anesthesiology and Surgery
University of Wisconsin Medical School
Madison, Wisconsin

KEVIN K. TREMPER, MD
Professor and Chairman
Department of Anesthesiology
University of Michigan Medical Center
Ann Arbor, Michigan

B. CRAIG WELDON, MD
Associate Professor
Department of Anesthesiology and Pediatrics
Duke University School of Medicine
Durham, North Carolina